INTRODUCTION

Brief Overview of ADHD and Autism

Attention-deficit/hyperactivity disorder (ADHD) and autism spectrum disorder (ASD) are two distinct neurodevelopmental conditions that affect individuals in different ways. While they are separate disorders, they can sometimes exhibit overlapping symptoms and challenges. Understanding the characteristics of each condition is crucial in order to provide appropriate support and interventions for individuals diagnosed with ADHD or ASD.

ADHD is a neurodevelopmental disorder characterized by persistent patterns of inattention, hyperactivity, and impulsivity that interfere with daily functioning and development. Individuals with ADHD often struggle with maintaining focus, organizing tasks, staying on track, and controlling impulsive behaviors. ADHD can manifest in childhood and persist into adulthood, impacting various aspects of life, including education, work, and relationships.

Autism spectrum disorder (ASD) is a complex developmental condition that affects social interaction, communication, and behavior. Individuals with ASD may have difficulties with social communication and interaction, such as understanding non-verbal cues or developing reciprocal relationships. They may also display repetitive behaviors, restricted interests, and sensory sensitivities. Autism is typically diagnosed in early childhood, but its impact can vary widely across individuals, ranging from mild to severe.

Both ADHD and ASD are considered neurodevelopmental conditions because they involve atypical brain development and functioning. While the exact causes are not fully understood, research suggests a combination of genetic, environmental, and neurological factors play a role in their development. It is important to note that ADHD and ASD are not a result of poor parenting or social circumstances, dispelling any misconceptions or stigma associated with these conditions.

Importance of Understanding and

Managing these Conditions

Understanding and effectively managing ADHD and ASD are crucial for several reasons. Firstly, individuals with these conditions often face unique challenges that can significantly impact their daily lives. By gaining knowledge about the specific characteristics and needs associated with ADHD and ASD, parents, educators, healthcare professionals, and society as a whole can provide appropriate support, accommodations, and interventions.

Importance of understanding ADHD:

1. **Recognition and early intervention:** Understanding ADHD allows for early recognition of symptoms, leading to timely intervention. Early diagnosis and intervention can help mitigate the negative effects of ADHD on academic performance, social interactions, and emotional well-being.

2. **Accommodations and support:** Understanding ADHD enables educators and parents to provide appropriate accommodations and support strategies to help individuals with ADHD succeed in academic settings. This may include modified teaching techniques, organizational tools, or behavioral interventions tailored to the individual's needs.

3. **Promoting self-awareness and self-advocacy:**

Knowledge about ADHD empowers individuals to understand their strengths, weaknesses, and unique learning styles. By promoting self-awareness and self-advocacy skills, individuals with ADHD can navigate their daily lives more effectively and advocate for their needs in various contexts.

Importance of understanding ASD:

1. **Early intervention and therapy:** Understanding ASD allows for early identification and intervention, which is critical for maximizing developmental outcomes. Early intervention services, such as behavioral therapy, speech therapy, and occupational therapy, can help individuals with ASD improve their communication, social skills, and adaptive behaviors.

2. **Creating inclusive environments:** Knowledge about ASD helps create inclusive environments that accommodate the unique sensory and communication needs of individuals with ASD. By understanding their strengths and challenges, educators, employers, and community members can foster acceptance, promote social inclusion, and reduce barriers to participation.

3. **Family support and community engagement:** Understanding ASD enables families to access support services and connect with other individuals and families who share similar experiences. Community engagement, such as participating in support groups or advocacy

organizations, can provide a sense of belonging and help families navigate the challenges associated with ASD.

Scope of the Guide

The guide aims to provide a comprehensive understanding of ADHD and ASD, addressing various aspects related to these conditions. It will cover topics such as:

1. **Definition and diagnostic criteria:** An overview of the diagnostic criteria and clinical guidelines used to identify and diagnose ADHD and ASD.

2. **Characteristics and symptoms:** A detailed exploration of the characteristic symptoms, behaviors, and challenges associated with ADHD and ASD.

3. **Causes and risk factors:** An examination of the potential causes and risk factors involved in the development of ADHD and ASD, including genetic and environmental influences.

4. **Diagnosis and assessment:** An overview of the diagnostic process, assessment tools, and professionals involved in diagnosing ADHD and ASD.

5. **Treatment and interventions:** A comprehensive exploration of evidence-based treatments, interventions, and therapies available for individuals with ADHD and ASD. This section will also address the importance of a multidisciplinary approach and the role of

various professionals in providing support.

6. **Support strategies and accommodations:** A discussion of practical strategies, accommodations, and modifications that can be implemented in educational, occupational, and social settings to support individuals with ADHD and ASD.

7. **Lifestyle and self-care:** An exploration of lifestyle factors, self-care practices, and coping strategies that can help individuals with ADHD and ASD manage their symptoms and enhance their overall well-being.

8. **Advocacy and community resources:** An overview of advocacy resources, support networks, and community organizations that can provide assistance, information, and opportunities for individuals and families affected by ADHD and ASD.

By addressing these topics, the guide aims to promote a deeper understanding of ADHD and ASD, foster inclusivity, and provide practical guidance for individuals, families, educators, healthcare professionals, and the broader community.

UNDERSTANDING ADHD

Attention-deficit/hyperactivity disorder (ADHD) is a neurodevelopmental disorder that affects both children and adults. It is characterized by persistent patterns of inattention, hyperactivity, and impulsivity that significantly impair daily functioning and quality of life.

1. Inattention: Individuals with ADHD often struggle with maintaining focus and sustaining attention, especially in tasks that require sustained mental effort or are not inherently stimulating. They may have difficulty organizing tasks and activities, often becoming easily distracted by external stimuli.

2. Hyperactivity: Hyperactivity is typically manifested as excessive and restless physical activity. Children with hyperactive ADHD may have difficulty remaining seated, constantly fidget or squirm, and display an inability to engage in quiet activities. In adults, hyperactivity may manifest as inner restlessness and a constant need to be busy.

3. Impulsivity: Impulsivity refers to acting without forethought or consideration of the consequences. People with ADHD may have difficulty inhibiting their immediate responses or interrupting others. They may engage in impulsive behaviors without considering the potential risks or long-term implications.

It's important to note that the severity and specific combination of these symptoms can vary among individuals with ADHD. Some individuals may predominantly exhibit symptoms of inattention, while others may primarily display hyperactivity and impulsivity. Additionally, the symptoms must be present in multiple settings, such as at home, school, or work, and have a negative impact on various aspects of life.

Types of ADHD (Inattentive, Hyperactive/ Impulsive, Combined)

ADHD can be classified into three subtypes: inattentive type, hyperactive/impulsive type, and combined type.

1. Inattentive Type: Individuals with the inattentive type of ADHD primarily struggle with inattention symptoms. They may have difficulty staying focused, following instructions, and organizing tasks. They may appear forgetful, easily distracted, and frequently lose track of their belongings. This type is often referred to as Attention-Deficit Disorder (ADD).

2. Hyperactive/Impulsive Type: The hyperactive/impulsive type of ADHD is characterized by prominent symptoms of hyperactivity and impulsivity. Individuals may be excessively restless, have difficulty staying seated, and engage in impulsive behaviors without thinking through the consequences. They may interrupt others frequently and struggle with patience and self-control.

3. Combined Type: The combined type of ADHD is the most common subtype, where individuals exhibit symptoms of both inattention and hyperactivity/impulsivity. They may struggle with maintaining focus, exhibit restlessness, and display impulsive behaviors.

This subtype often presents with the most significant impairments across multiple areas of life.

The diagnosis of the specific subtype is based on the predominant symptoms observed and their impact on daily functioning.

Common Symptoms and Their Impact on Daily Life

ADHD symptoms can have a significant impact on various aspects of daily life, including education, work, relationships, and overall well-being.

1. **Academic Challenges:** Children with ADHD often face difficulties in school. They may struggle to pay attention in class, leading to decreased academic performance. Poor organizational skills and forgetfulness can result in missed assignments or incomplete tasks. These challenges can affect self-esteem and hinder educational progress.

2. **Impaired Work Performance:** Adults with ADHD may experience difficulties in the workplace. Inattention can lead to decreased productivity and difficulties meeting deadlines. Impulsivity and poor impulse control may affect

decision-making and lead to impulsive job changes or conflicts with colleagues.

3. Relationship Issues: The symptoms of ADHD can strain relationships. Inattentiveness and forgetfulness may cause frustration and misunderstandings with partners, friends, and family members. Impulsivity can lead to impulsive or reckless behavior that affects interpersonal dynamics and the ability to maintain long-term relationships.

4. Emotional and Psychological Impact: ADHD can contribute to emotional and psychological challenges. Individuals may experience frustration, low self-esteem, and a sense of underachievement due to difficulties managing symptoms. The chronic stress of dealing with ADHD-related impairments can also contribute to anxiety and depression.

Addressing these challenges often requires a comprehensive approach involving behavioral interventions, psychoeducation, and, in some cases, medication.

Causes and Risk Factors

The exact causes of ADHD are not yet fully understood, but research suggests a combination of genetic, neurobiological, and environmental factors.

1. Genetic Factors: ADHD tends to run in families, indicating a genetic component. Studies have identified specific genes associated with the disorder, although the exact genetic mechanisms are still being investigated. Having a close family member with ADHD increases the risk of developing the disorder.

2. Neurobiological Factors: Brain imaging studies have revealed differences in the brain structure and functioning of individuals with ADHD. Reduced volume in certain brain regions involved in attention, impulse control, and executive functions has been observed. Neurotransmitter imbalances, particularly involving dopamine and norepinephrine, may also contribute to ADHD symptoms.

3. Environmental Factors: Prenatal and early-life factors can influence the risk of developing ADHD. Exposure to tobacco smoke, alcohol, or drugs during pregnancy, premature birth, low birth weight, and lead exposure have been associated with an increased likelihood of ADHD.

Additionally, high levels of stress in the family or a chaotic home environment may contribute to the development of ADHD symptoms.

It's important to note that ADHD is a complex disorder, and no single cause or risk factor can fully explain its development. Rather, it is likely a combination of genetic and environmental factors interacting with each other.

Diagnosis Process

Diagnosing ADHD involves a comprehensive assessment that considers the individual's symptoms, history, and observations from multiple settings. The process typically involves the following steps:

1. **Clinical Interview:** A healthcare professional conducts a detailed interview with the individual and, if applicable, their parents or caregivers. They gather information about the individual's symptoms, developmental history, and the impact of ADHD on different areas of life.

2. **Rating Scales and Questionnaires:** Standardized rating scales and questionnaires are often used to assess ADHD symptoms and their severity. These may be completed

by the individual, parents, teachers, or other relevant individuals familiar with the person's behavior in different settings.

3. Medical Examination: A thorough medical examination is conducted to rule out any underlying medical conditions or medications that could be causing or exacerbating ADHD-like symptoms. It also helps identify any comorbidities that may be present.

4. Diagnostic Criteria: The healthcare professional compares the individual's symptoms and functional impairments to the criteria outlined in the Diagnostic and Statistical Manual of Mental Disorders (DSM-5), a widely used diagnostic reference.

5. Multimodal Assessment: In some cases, additional assessments may be conducted to evaluate cognitive functioning, executive functions, and academic or occupational performance. These assessments provide a comprehensive understanding of the individual's strengths and weaknesses.

The diagnosis of ADHD is complex and requires a careful

evaluation by a qualified healthcare professional with expertise in neurodevelopmental disorders.

Associated Conditions and Comorbidities

ADHD is often associated with several other conditions and comorbidities, meaning they frequently occur together in individuals. Common comorbidities include:

1. Learning Disabilities: Individuals with ADHD often have specific learning difficulties, such as dyslexia or dyscalculia. These learning disabilities can further impact academic performance and require targeted interventions.

2. Oppositional Defiant Disorder (ODD) and Conduct Disorder (CD): ODD and CD are behavioral disorders that commonly co-occur with ADHD. ODD involves a pattern of defiant, disobedient, and hostile behavior, while CD involves more severe antisocial behaviors, such as aggression and violation of rules.

3. Anxiety and Depression: ADHD increases the risk of developing anxiety disorders and depression. The challenges associated with managing ADHD symptoms, coping with daily impairments, and facing social difficulties can contribute to these co-occurring mental health conditions.

4. Autism Spectrum Disorder (ASD): ADHD and ASD commonly coexist. While they are distinct conditions, they share overlapping symptoms, such as difficulties with social interactions and executive functions. Accurate diagnosis and differentiation between the two are crucial for appropriate intervention.

5. Substance Use Disorders: Individuals with ADHD have an increased vulnerability to substance use disorders. Impulsivity, sensation-seeking behavior, and difficulties with self-regulation contribute to a higher risk of substance abuse and addiction.

It's important to address these comorbid conditions alongside ADHD to ensure comprehensive treatment and support for individuals affected by multiple disorders.

In conclusion, ADHD is a neurodevelopmental disorder characterized by inattention, hyperactivity, and impulsivity. It can manifest in different subtypes and has a significant impact on various aspects of daily life. The causes of ADHD involve a complex interplay of genetic, neurobiological, and environmental factors. The diagnosis process involves a comprehensive assessment, and ADHD commonly co-occurs with other conditions, emphasizing the need for a multidimensional approach to treatment and support.

UNDERSTANDING AUTISM

Definition and Characteristics of Autism Spectrum Disorder (ASD)

Autism Spectrum Disorder (ASD) is a neurodevelopmental disorder that affects individuals in various ways, primarily impacting social communication, behavior, and sensory processing. It is characterized by a wide range of symptoms and severity levels, leading to the term "spectrum." ASD is typically diagnosed in early childhood, although some individuals may receive a diagnosis later in life.

The core characteristics of ASD include:

1. **Impairments in social interaction:** Individuals with ASD may struggle with understanding and appropriately responding to social cues, such as facial expressions, gestures, and body

language. They may have difficulty establishing and maintaining relationships, interpreting others' emotions, and engaging in reciprocal conversation.

2. **Communication difficulties:** Many individuals with ASD experience challenges in verbal and non-verbal communication. They may have delayed language development, difficulty initiating or sustaining conversations, and a tendency to take language literally. Some individuals may use alternative forms of communication, such as sign language or augmentative and alternative communication (AAC) devices.

3. **Restricted interests and repetitive behaviors:** People with ASD often engage in repetitive behaviors or have intense, narrow interests. They may exhibit repetitive body movements (e.g., hand flapping, rocking), adherence to strict routines or rituals, and a strong resistance to change. They may also show a preoccupation with specific topics or objects.

4. **Sensory sensitivities:** Many individuals with ASD are hypersensitive or hyposensitive to sensory input. They may be highly sensitive to sounds, lights, textures, tastes, or smells, leading to sensory overload or avoidance. Alternatively, some individuals may seek sensory stimulation, such as by repeatedly touching or sniffing objects.

It is important to note that the manifestation and severity

of these characteristics can vary widely among individuals with ASD. Some may have mild symptoms and excel in specific areas, while others may have more significant challenges that impact multiple aspects of their lives.

Autism Severity Levels

To provide a clearer understanding of the range and impact of symptoms, clinicians often use severity levels to describe the functional limitations associated with ASD. These levels are based on the amount of support an individual requires to navigate daily life:

1. **Level 1 (Requiring support):** Individuals with Level 1 ASD, often referred to as "mild ASD," require some support to function in social situations. They may experience difficulties with social interactions and communication but can typically manage daily routines with minimal assistance.

2. **Level 2 (Requiring substantial support):** Individuals with Level 2 ASD, classified as "moderate ASD," have more pronounced social communication challenges. They may require substantial support to navigate social situations, transitions, and changes in routine. Their restricted interests and repetitive behaviors may interfere with functioning independently.

3. **Level 3 (Requiring very substantial support):**

Individuals with Level 3 ASD, considered "severe ASD," experience significant impairments in social communication and behavior. They require extensive support across all areas of daily life, including self-care, academic or work-related tasks, and social interactions.

These severity levels provide a framework for understanding the overall functional impact of ASD but should not be seen as fixed categories. Each individual with ASD is unique, and their support needs can change over time based on various factors, including intervention, therapy, and personal development.

Common Symptoms and Their Impact on Daily Life

The symptoms of ASD can significantly impact an individual's daily life across various domains:

1. **Social interactions:** Difficulties in social interaction can lead to challenges in forming and maintaining relationships, making friends, and understanding social norms and expectations. This can result in social isolation, feelings of loneliness, and a sense of being misunderstood.

2. **Communication:** Communication difficulties may hinder verbal and non-verbal expression, affecting an individual's ability to convey thoughts, needs, and emotions effectively. This

can lead to frustration, anxiety, and difficulty participating in academic, occupational, and social settings.

3. **Routines and flexibility:** People with ASD often rely on routines and sameness to navigate their environment. Any disruption or change to their established routines can cause significant distress and anxiety. Adapting to new situations, transitions, or unexpected events may require additional support and careful planning.

4. **Sensory sensitivities:** Individuals with ASD may experience sensory sensitivities that make certain sounds, sights, textures, or smells overwhelming or aversive. This can result in sensory overload, avoidance of specific environments or activities, and difficulties focusing or engaging in tasks that require sensory processing.

5. **Restricted interests and repetitive behaviors:** The presence of restricted interests and repetitive behaviors can consume a significant amount of time and attention, potentially interfering with daily routines, social interactions, and engagement in other activities. However, these interests can also provide a source of motivation and enjoyment for individuals with ASD.

Understanding and accommodating these symptoms is essential to help individuals with ASD thrive. By providing appropriate support, interventions, and accommodations, it is possible to enhance their quality of life, promote their independence, and facilitate their participation in various settings.

Causes and Risk Factors

The exact causes of ASD are not yet fully understood. However, research suggests that a combination of genetic, environmental, and neurological factors contribute to its development. Some known factors associated with an increased risk of ASD include:

1. **Genetic factors:** There is evidence of a genetic component in ASD. Certain gene mutations, chromosomal abnormalities, and a family history of ASD increase the likelihood of an individual developing the disorder. However, it is important to note that ASD is a complex condition with multiple genetic factors involved.

2. **Prenatal and early development:** Some prenatal and early developmental factors have been associated with an increased risk of ASD. These include maternal infections during pregnancy, certain prenatal medications, complications during birth, and low birth weight. However, it is important to note that these factors are not determinants and do not account for all cases of ASD.

3. **Neurological differences:** Neurological differences in brain structure and functioning have been observed in individuals with ASD.

These differences may affect the development of social communication and behavior regulation, contributing to the core symptoms of the disorder.

It is important to emphasize that ASD is not caused by parenting practices or social circumstances. Debunking such misconceptions is crucial in promoting understanding, reducing stigma, and supporting individuals and families affected by ASD.

Diagnosis Process

The diagnosis of ASD involves a comprehensive evaluation that considers an individual's developmental history, observed behaviors, and standardized assessment tools. The diagnostic process typically includes the following steps:

1. **Screening:** Healthcare providers may administer developmental screening tools during routine check-ups to identify any early signs of ASD. These screenings help determine if further evaluation is necessary.

2. **Comprehensive assessment:** A comprehensive assessment involves gathering information from multiple sources, including parents, caregivers, teachers, and healthcare professionals. It includes a thorough review of the individual's

developmental history, behavioral observations, and assessments of social communication, cognitive abilities, and adaptive functioning.

3. **Diagnostic criteria:** The evaluation is based on established diagnostic criteria, such as the Diagnostic and Statistical Manual of Mental Disorders (DSM-5) or the International Classification of Diseases (ICD-11). These criteria outline the specific symptoms and impairments that must be present for a diagnosis of ASD.

4. **Multidisciplinary approach:** The diagnostic process often involves a multidisciplinary team, including psychologists, psychiatrists, pediatricians, speech-language pathologists, and occupational therapists. Collaboration among professionals with expertise in ASD ensures a comprehensive assessment and accurate diagnosis.

5. **Differential diagnosis:** The evaluation also considers other conditions with similar symptoms to rule out alternative explanations for the observed behaviors. This helps ensure an accurate and specific diagnosis.

It is important to note that the diagnostic process may vary based on the age of the individual and the resources available in different regions. Early identification and diagnosis are crucial for early intervention and support, enabling individuals with ASD to access appropriate services and interventions.

Associated Conditions and Comorbidities

ASD is often associated with other conditions and comorbidities, meaning they coexist or occur alongside ASD. Some common associated conditions include:

1. **Intellectual disability:** Intellectual disability, characterized by limitations in intellectual functioning and adaptive behaviors, is seen in a subset of individuals with ASD. The severity of intellectual disability can vary widely.

2. **Attention-deficit/hyperactivity disorder (ADHD):** ADHD commonly co-occurs with ASD. Individuals with both ASD and ADHD may exhibit symptoms of inattention, hyperactivity, and impulsivity that further impact their daily functioning.

3. **Anxiety and depression:** People with ASD may experience higher rates of anxiety disorders and depression compared to the general population. These conditions can stem from difficulties with social interactions, communication challenges, and sensory sensitivities.

4. **Epilepsy:** Epilepsy, a neurological disorder characterized by recurrent seizures, is more prevalent in individuals with ASD compared to the general population. The relationship between ASD and epilepsy is complex and not yet fully understood.

5. **Sleep disturbances:** Sleep difficulties, such as

insomnia or irregular sleep patterns, are common among individuals with ASD. These sleep disturbances can further impact daily functioning and overall well-being.

Recognizing and addressing these associated conditions and comorbidities is important for providing comprehensive support and intervention strategies tailored to the individual's needs. A holistic approach that considers the full range of challenges and coexisting conditions can significantly improve outcomes for individuals with ASD.

OVERLAPPING TRAITS AND DIFFERENTIATING FEATURES

Similarities and Differences between ADHD and Autism

ADHD and Autism Spectrum Disorder (ASD) are two distinct neurodevelopmental conditions with overlapping symptoms. While they share some similarities, they also have distinct characteristics:

Similarities:

1. **Executive functioning difficulties:** Both ADHD and ASD can involve challenges with executive functioning, which includes skills such as attention, organization, planning, and impulse control. Difficulties in these areas can affect academic performance, daily routines, and social

interactions.

2. **Sensory sensitivities:** Both conditions commonly involve sensory sensitivities. Individuals with ADHD and ASD may be hypersensitive or hyposensitive to certain sounds, sights, textures, tastes, or smells, which can impact their comfort and functioning in sensory-rich environments.

Differences:

1. **Social communication and interaction:** While social difficulties are present in both ADHD and ASD, the nature of these challenges differs. In ASD, the impairment in social communication and interaction is a core feature, characterized by difficulties in understanding social cues, maintaining relationships, and interpreting emotions. In ADHD, social difficulties are often secondary to impulsivity, inattention, or hyperactivity.

2. **Repetitive behaviors and restricted interests:** Individuals with ASD commonly exhibit repetitive behaviors and intense, narrow interests, which are not prominent features of ADHD. These behaviors may include repetitive body movements, adherence to routines, and a strong attachment to specific objects or topics. In ADHD, impulsivity, hyperactivity, and inattention are the primary characteristics.

3. **Hyperactivity and impulsivity:** Hyperactivity and impulsivity are more prominent in ADHD

compared to ASD. Individuals with ADHD often struggle with excessive movement, restlessness, and impulsive behaviors, whereas individuals with ASD may exhibit more repetitive movements or a tendency to be highly focused on specific activities or interests.

4. **Language development:** Language delays or impairments are more commonly associated with ASD than ADHD. While individuals with ADHD may experience difficulties in language production or processing, the severity and pattern of language impairments are typically more pronounced in ASD.

It is important to recognize these similarities and differences to ensure accurate diagnosis and appropriate interventions for individuals who may exhibit overlapping traits.

Coexistence of ADHD and Autism

ADHD and ASD can coexist in some individuals, leading to a dual diagnosis. The presence of both conditions can present additional challenges and complexities. Research suggests a high rate of comorbidity between ADHD and ASD, with estimates ranging from 30% to 80%.

When ADHD and ASD coexist, it can result in a more complex clinical presentation and potentially exacerbate the challenges associated with each condition. The coexistence may impact social interactions, attentional regulation, impulse control, and adaptive functioning.

Individuals with both ADHD and ASD may require a comprehensive and tailored approach to intervention that addresses the specific needs associated with each condition. Collaborative efforts among healthcare professionals, educators, and families are essential to develop an individualized support plan that considers the unique strengths and challenges of the individual.

Challenges in Accurate Diagnosis and Differentiation

Accurately diagnosing ADHD and ASD, and differentiating between the two, can be challenging due to several factors:

1. **Overlapping symptoms:** Both conditions share some common symptoms, such as difficulties with attention, executive functioning, and social interactions. These overlapping symptoms can make it difficult to determine the primary diagnosis or recognize the presence of both conditions.

2. **Variability in symptom presentation:** The symptoms of ADHD and ASD can manifest differently in each individual, leading to

variability in symptom presentation. This individual variation can complicate the diagnostic process and contribute to the challenges in accurate differentiation.

3. **Comorbidity and shared risk factors:** ADHD and ASD often coexist with other conditions, such as anxiety, depression, or intellectual disabilities. These comorbidities can further complicate the diagnostic process and make it challenging to attribute specific symptoms to a single condition.

4. **Developmental changes:** Symptoms of ADHD and ASD can evolve and change over time, particularly in early childhood. Some symptoms may become more apparent or recede, further adding complexity to the diagnostic process.

To overcome these challenges and achieve an accurate diagnosis, a comprehensive evaluation is necessary. This evaluation should involve input from multiple sources, including parents, teachers, and healthcare professionals. A thorough assessment of the individual's developmental history, observed behaviors, and standardized assessment tools can help identify the primary diagnosis and determine the presence of any coexisting conditions.

Strategies to Identify Overlapping Traits

To identify overlapping traits and differentiate between ADHD and ASD, the following strategies can be helpful:

1. **Comprehensive evaluation:** A comprehensive evaluation conducted by professionals experienced in diagnosing and treating neurodevelopmental conditions is crucial. This evaluation should include a thorough assessment of behavioral observations, developmental history, cognitive abilities, social communication, and executive functioning.

2. **Observation across settings:** It is important to gather information about the individual's behavior and functioning in different settings, such as home, school, and community. This can provide a more comprehensive understanding of how symptoms manifest in various contexts.

3. **Collaboration among professionals:** Collaboration among professionals from different disciplines, such as psychologists, psychiatrists, speech-language pathologists, and occupational therapists, is essential. Their expertise and diverse perspectives can contribute to a more accurate diagnosis and differentiation.

4. **Longitudinal assessment:** Tracking and monitoring symptoms over time can provide valuable information for differentiation. Examining the stability and persistence of certain symptoms and their impact on functioning can aid in understanding the underlying condition.

5. **Consideration of comorbidities:** Recognizing and addressing comorbidities is essential. Thorough assessment and consideration of the presence of other conditions, such as anxiety or intellectual disabilities, can help determine their contribution

to the overall presentation.

By utilizing a multidimensional approach and considering the individual's unique profile of strengths and challenges, healthcare professionals can work together to identify overlapping traits, differentiate between ADHD and ASD, and provide appropriate support and interventions tailored to the individual's needs.

MANAGING ADHD AND AUTISM

Early Intervention and Support

Early intervention plays a crucial role in the management of ADHD and Autism Spectrum Disorder (ASD). Timely identification and intervention can help address challenges, promote development, and improve outcomes. Key aspects of early intervention and support include:

1. **Screening and assessment:** Early identification involves the use of screening tools to identify early signs of ADHD or ASD. If a concern is raised, a comprehensive assessment is conducted to determine the presence and severity of the condition.

2. **Parent education and training:** Providing parents with information and resources about ADHD and ASD empowers them to understand their child's needs, access appropriate services, and implement effective strategies at home.

3. **Early developmental interventions:** Early interventions focus on promoting developmental milestones, enhancing communication skills,

and supporting social interactions. These interventions may include speech and language therapy, occupational therapy, and developmental play-based interventions.

4. **Individualized intervention plans:** Each child's needs are unique, and intervention plans should be tailored accordingly. Collaborating with a team of professionals, including therapists, educators, and healthcare providers, ensures a comprehensive and individualized approach.

5. **Supportive services:** Access to supportive services, such as counseling, support groups, and community resources, can provide emotional support and guidance for families navigating the challenges associated with ADHD and ASD.

Early intervention aims to provide children and families with the tools and support necessary to maximize their potential and enhance their quality of life.

Behavioral and Educational Interventions

Behavioral and educational interventions are widely used to support individuals with ADHD and ASD. These interventions focus on addressing specific symptoms, promoting skill development, and improving adaptive behaviors. Some commonly used interventions include:

1. Applied Behavior Analysis (ABA):

ABA is a therapeutic approach that uses principles of learning and behavior to bring about positive changes. It involves breaking down complex skills into smaller achievable steps and using reinforcement techniques to encourage desired behaviors while reducing challenging behaviors.

2. Social Skills Training:

Social skills training aims to enhance social interactions, communication, and relationship-building abilities. It involves teaching individuals with ADHD or ASD how to recognize social cues, engage in conversations, and develop appropriate social behaviors.

3. Cognitive-Behavioral Therapy (CBT):

CBT is a form of psychotherapy that focuses on identifying and changing unhelpful thoughts and behaviors. It can be beneficial for individuals with ADHD or ASD by targeting specific challenges, such as managing impulsivity, improving organizational skills, or reducing anxiety.

These interventions are typically implemented in various

settings, including schools, clinics, and homes, with the involvement of trained professionals.

Medication Options and Considerations

Medication can be an important component of treatment for individuals with ADHD or ASD. However, it is crucial to note that medication is not appropriate or necessary for everyone, and the decision to use medication should be made in collaboration with healthcare professionals. Considerations include:

1. **Stimulant medication (e.g., methylphenidate, amphetamines):** Stimulant medications are commonly prescribed for ADHD. They can help improve attention, impulse control, and hyperactivity. However, they may have side effects, and regular monitoring is essential.

2. **Non-stimulant medication (e.g., atomoxetine, guanfacine):** Non-stimulant medications are an alternative for individuals who do not respond well to or cannot tolerate stimulant medications. These medications can help improve attention and impulse control.

It is important to work closely with a healthcare professional to determine the most appropriate medication option, monitor effectiveness, and manage any potential side effects.

Parenting and Family Support

Parenting and family support are integral to the well-being and development of children with ADHD or ASD. Some strategies for parents and families include:

1. **Education and understanding:** Learning about ADHD or ASD helps parents better understand their child's challenges, strengths, and needs. Education can empower parents to advocate for their child, access appropriate services, and implement effective strategies at home.

2. **Structured routines and consistency:** Establishing consistent routines and providing structure can help children with ADHD or ASD navigate daily tasks and transitions more effectively. Clear expectations, visual schedules, and consistent rules can promote a sense of predictability and reduce anxiety.

3. **Positive reinforcement and rewards:** Using positive reinforcement techniques, such as praise, rewards, or token systems, can encourage desired behaviors and motivate children to make positive choices.

4. **Self-care and support:** Taking care of oneself is crucial for parents and caregivers. Seeking support from professionals, joining support groups, and practicing self-care activities can help manage stress and enhance overall well-being.

Supportive and nurturing family environments

significantly contribute to the success and overall development of children with ADHD or ASD.

School Accommodations and Individualized Education Programs (IEPs)

Schools play a vital role in supporting students with ADHD or ASD. Accommodations and Individualized Education Programs (IEPs) can be established to meet their unique needs. Some strategies include:

1. **Modifications to the learning environment:** Providing a structured and predictable classroom environment, minimizing distractions, and creating visual supports can benefit students with ADHD or ASD.

2. **Individualized instruction:** Tailoring teaching strategies and materials to match the student's learning style and strengths can enhance engagement and comprehension.

3. **Behavior management strategies:** Implementing behavior management techniques, such as token systems, visual schedules, or designated quiet areas, can help students with ADHD or ASD stay focused and manage their behavior.

4. **Social skills support:** Offering social skills training or facilitating peer interactions can foster social growth and inclusion for students with ADHD or ASD.

Collaboration among teachers, parents, and specialized support staff is essential to create effective IEPs and ensure the successful implementation of accommodations in the school setting.

Supportive Therapies and Alternative Treatments

In addition to traditional interventions, some individuals may benefit from supportive therapies and alternative treatments. These can complement other interventions and address specific needs. Some examples include:

1. **Speech and language therapy:** Speech and language therapy can help individuals improve communication skills, including speech articulation, language comprehension, and social communication.

2. **Occupational therapy:** Occupational therapy focuses on developing skills necessary for daily activities and promoting independence. It can address sensory sensitivities, fine motor skills, self-regulation, and adaptive behaviors.

3. **Dietary interventions:** Some individuals with ADHD or ASD may benefit from dietary modifications, such as eliminating certain food additives or following specific nutritional plans. It is important to consult with healthcare professionals or dieticians before making any

significant dietary changes.

4. **Mindfulness and relaxation techniques:** Mindfulness practices, deep breathing exercises, and relaxation techniques can help individuals with ADHD or ASD manage stress, improve self-regulation, and enhance overall well-being.

While these supportive therapies and alternative treatments may have varying levels of evidence supporting their effectiveness, it is crucial to consult with professionals and consider individual needs and preferences before incorporating them into a treatment plan.

In conclusion, a comprehensive approach to intervention and support for individuals with ADHD or ASD includes early identification, behavioral and educational interventions, medication considerations, parenting and family support, school accommodations, and access to supportive therapies. By addressing the unique needs of individuals and providing a multidimensional approach, we can promote their development, well-being, and overall quality of life.

STRATEGIES FOR DAILY LIFE

Organization and Time Management Tips

Organization and time management can significantly improve the daily functioning of individuals with ADHD or ASD. Here are some tips to promote organization and effective time management:

1. **Establish routines and schedules:** Create structured daily routines and schedules that include specific times for tasks, activities, and breaks. Consistency and predictability can help individuals with ADHD or ASD stay organized and manage their time more effectively.

2. **Use visual aids:** Visual supports, such as calendars, to-do lists, or visual schedules, can be valuable tools for organization. These visual aids provide a visual representation of tasks and help individuals understand and remember their daily responsibilities.

3. **Break tasks into smaller steps:** Large tasks can be overwhelming, making it difficult for individuals to get started. Breaking tasks into smaller, more manageable steps allows for a clearer focus and a

sense of progress as each step is completed.

4. **Set reminders and use alarms:** Utilize technology, such as smartphones or electronic devices, to set reminders and alarms for important tasks, appointments, or deadlines. This can help individuals with ADHD or ASD stay on track and manage their time effectively.

5. **Organize physical spaces:** Maintaining an organized physical environment can reduce visual and sensory distractions. Utilize storage systems, labels, and clear spaces to enhance organization and minimize clutter.

6. **Prioritize tasks:** Teach individuals how to prioritize tasks based on importance and urgency. Identifying and tackling high-priority tasks first can prevent procrastination and reduce stress.

Remember, everyone's organizational needs are unique, so it is essential to adapt these strategies to suit individual preferences and abilities.

Effective Communication and Social Skills Development

Effective communication and social skills development are crucial for individuals with ADHD or ASD to build and maintain meaningful relationships. Here are some strategies to enhance communication and social skills:

1. **Teach active listening:** Encourage individuals to practice active listening skills, such as maintaining eye contact, nodding, and paraphrasing what others say. This helps improve understanding and shows respect for the speaker.

2. **Practice turn-taking:** Teach the concept of turn-taking during conversations to ensure equal participation. Encourage individuals to wait their turn, listen attentively, and respond appropriately.

3. **Use visual supports:** Visual supports, like social stories, picture cues, or visual schedules, can help individuals with ADHD or ASD understand social expectations and navigate social situations more effectively.

4. **Model and teach non-verbal cues:** Non-verbal cues, such as facial expressions, body language, and tone of voice, are important for understanding and conveying emotions. Help individuals recognize and interpret these cues to improve social interactions.

5. **Role-play and practice social scenarios:** Engage individuals in role-playing activities to practice social skills in a safe and supportive environment. This can help them build confidence, improve their understanding of social norms, and develop problem-solving strategies.

6. **Encourage perspective-taking:** Foster empathy and perspective-taking skills by encouraging individuals to consider others' feelings and viewpoints. This promotes understanding,

respect, and effective communication.

7. **Provide social skills training:** Consider enrolling individuals in structured social skills training programs or groups where they can learn and practice social skills alongside peers.

Remember, social skills development is an ongoing process, and patience and reinforcement are key. Consistency and opportunities for practice in real-life social situations are essential for progress.

Coping with Sensory Sensitivities

Individuals with ADHD or ASD often experience sensory sensitivities that can be overwhelming and affect daily functioning. Here are strategies to help cope with sensory sensitivities:

1. **Identify triggers:** Recognize specific sensory triggers that can cause discomfort or overwhelm. These triggers may include certain sounds, textures, lights, or smells. Once identified, individuals can take steps to minimize or avoid these triggers whenever possible.

2. **Provide sensory breaks:** Allow individuals to take sensory breaks when they feel overwhelmed. This can involve retreating to a quiet space, engaging in calming activities, or using sensory tools like fidget toys or weighted blankets to provide comfort and regulation.

3. **Create a sensory-friendly environment:** Make adjustments to the physical environment to accommodate sensory sensitivities. This can include using dimmer lighting, reducing background noise, or providing comfortable seating options.

4. **Use sensory integration techniques:** Engage in sensory integration activities that can help regulate sensory input. These activities can include deep pressure activities, rhythmic movements, or sensory diets designed in collaboration with occupational therapists.

5. **Gradual exposure:** Gradually expose individuals to sensory stimuli that may be challenging. Start with low-intensity exposure and gradually increase the level of sensory input to desensitize and build tolerance over time.

6. **Communication and self-advocacy:** Encourage individuals to communicate their sensory sensitivities to others and advocate for their needs. This can involve using clear and assertive communication to express discomfort or requesting reasonable accommodations.

By understanding and addressing sensory sensitivities, individuals with ADHD or ASD can better manage their sensory experiences and reduce associated stress and anxiety.

Stress Management and Relaxation Techniques

Stress management and relaxation techniques are essential for individuals with ADHD or ASD to reduce anxiety and promote overall well-being. Here are some strategies to consider:

1. **Deep breathing exercises:** Teach deep breathing techniques, such as diaphragmatic breathing or box breathing, to help individuals calm their bodies and minds. Deep breathing can be practiced in various settings to reduce stress and promote relaxation.

2. **Mindfulness and meditation:** Introduce mindfulness practices to help individuals stay present, increase self-awareness, and manage stress. Mindfulness exercises, such as body scans or guided meditations, can promote relaxation and emotional regulation.

3. **Physical exercise:** Encourage regular physical exercise, as it can help reduce stress, improve mood, and increase overall well-being. Activities such as walking, biking, swimming, or participating in sports can be beneficial.

4. **Hobbies and creative outlets:** Engage individuals in activities they enjoy and find relaxing, such as drawing, painting, playing musical instruments, or engaging in crafts. These activities provide an outlet for self-expression and promote stress relief.

5. **Time for self-care:** Emphasize the importance of self-care activities, such as taking breaks,

engaging in hobbies, practicing relaxation techniques, or spending time in nature. Encourage individuals to prioritize self-care as part of their daily routine.

6. **Healthy lifestyle habits:** Promote healthy lifestyle habits, including a balanced diet, regular sleep patterns, and maintaining social connections. These factors contribute to overall well-being and stress reduction.

Remember, it is essential to tailor stress management techniques to individual preferences and needs. Regular practice and incorporating these strategies into daily routines can lead to increased resilience and better stress management skills.

Building Resilience and Self-Advocacy Skills

Building resilience and self-advocacy skills empower individuals with ADHD or ASD to navigate challenges and advocate for their needs. Here are strategies to promote resilience and self-advocacy:

1. **Foster a growth mindset:** Encourage individuals to adopt a growth mindset, viewing challenges as opportunities for learning and growth. Teach them to approach setbacks with perseverance and adaptability.

2. **Identify strengths and interests:** Help individuals recognize and celebrate their unique

strengths and interests. Focusing on strengths can boost confidence and resilience in overcoming challenges.

3. **Encourage problem-solving skills:** Teach problem-solving strategies, such as breaking problems into smaller parts, brainstorming solutions, and evaluating the pros and cons of different options. This equips individuals to tackle challenges independently.

4. **Develop self-advocacy skills:** Teach individuals to identify their needs, communicate them effectively, and seek appropriate support and accommodations. Encourage them to actively participate in decision-making processes that affect their lives.

5. **Promote self-reflection:** Encourage individuals to reflect on their experiences, emotions, and strategies that work well for them. This self-reflection enhances self-awareness and helps identify effective coping mechanisms.

6. **Build a support network:** Help individuals develop a supportive network of friends, family, teachers, or mentors who can provide encouragement, guidance, and understanding.

7. **Celebrate progress:** Recognize and celebrate achievements, both big and small. This reinforces resilience and self-confidence.

By fostering resilience and self-advocacy skills, individuals with ADHD or ASD can develop the confidence and abilities to overcome challenges and achieve their goals.

Navigating Transitions and Changes

Transitions and changes can be challenging for individuals with ADHD or ASD due to difficulties with flexibility and adapting to new situations. Here are strategies to help navigate transitions effectively:

1. **Prepare in advance:** Provide individuals with information and preparation for upcoming transitions or changes. This can include discussing what to expect, showing visual supports or social stories, or creating a transition plan.

2. **Establish routines:** Maintain consistent routines during times of change to provide stability and predictability. Routines can serve as anchors and help individuals feel more comfortable in new or uncertain situations.

3. **Use visual supports:** Utilize visual schedules, calendars, or checklists to visually represent transitions and changes. These supports can provide a clear understanding of what is happening and what to expect next.

4. **Provide transition warnings:** Offer warnings or countdowns before transitions occur. This gives individuals time to mentally prepare and adjust their focus from one activity to the next.

5. **Use social narratives:** Create social narratives that explain the purpose and expectations of a

transition or change. These narratives can help individuals understand the reasons behind the transition and reduce anxiety.

6. **Offer support during transitions:** Provide support and guidance during transitions, particularly when individuals may struggle with organization or navigating new environments. Offer assistance in managing tasks, finding resources, or adjusting to new routines.

7. **Encourage self-regulation strategies:** Teach individuals self-regulation techniques, such as deep breathing or positive self-talk, that can be used during transitions to manage anxiety or frustration.

Remember, patience, flexibility, and understanding are key when supporting individuals with ADHD or ASD through transitions. Gradual exposure and consistent support can help them navigate changes more smoothly.

SUPPORTING NEURODIVERSE INDIVIDUALS

Understanding Neurodiversity

Neurodiversity is a concept that recognizes and embraces the natural variations in human neurological functioning. It highlights that neurodiverse individuals, including those with ADHD or Autism Spectrum Disorder (ASD), have unique strengths, perspectives, and ways of experiencing the world. Understanding neurodiversity is essential for promoting inclusivity, acceptance, and creating supportive environments. Here's an overview of key aspects related to neurodiversity:

1. **Neurodiversity as a spectrum:** Neurodiversity encompasses a broad range of neurological differences, including but not limited to ADHD and ASD. These differences can manifest in various ways, impacting individuals' cognitive, sensory, social, or emotional functioning.

Recognizing neurodiversity as a spectrum emphasizes that each person's experience is unique.

2. **Strengths-based approach:** Embracing neurodiversity means valuing the strengths and abilities of neurodiverse individuals. Rather than focusing solely on deficits or challenges, it is important to recognize and nurture their exceptional skills, talents, and unique perspectives. This strengths-based approach promotes self-confidence and self-esteem.

3. **Respecting neurodiverse perspectives:** Neurodiversity challenges the notion of a "normal" or "typical" neurology. It encourages society to appreciate and respect different ways of thinking, learning, and perceiving the world. By embracing diverse perspectives, we foster creativity, innovation, and problem-solving.

4. **Rejecting pathologization:** Neurodiversity advocates argue against pathologizing neurodiverse individuals and instead emphasize the need to understand and accept neurological differences as natural variations of human diversity. This perspective promotes a shift away from viewing neurodiverse traits as disorders or deficits.

Promoting Inclusivity and Acceptance

Promoting inclusivity and acceptance is crucial in creating a supportive and inclusive environment for neurodiverse individuals. By fostering understanding and embracing diversity, we can ensure that everyone feels valued and respected. Here are some strategies for promoting inclusivity and acceptance:

1. **Education and awareness:** Increase awareness and understanding of neurodiversity through education and information-sharing. Provide resources, workshops, and training sessions to educate individuals about different neurological profiles and the strengths of neurodiverse individuals.

2. **Encourage empathy and understanding:** Foster empathy and understanding by promoting open dialogue and discussions about neurodiversity. Encourage individuals to listen, ask questions, and learn from the experiences of neurodiverse individuals and their families.

3. **Create inclusive environments:** Ensure that environments at home, school, and work are designed to be inclusive and accommodating. Make reasonable accommodations to support neurodiverse individuals in their daily activities, learning, and work settings.

4. **Promote diversity in media and representation:** Encourage accurate and positive representation of neurodiverse individuals in the media, literature, and other forms of communication. This helps challenge stereotypes and promotes inclusivity in society.

5. **Encourage peer support and advocacy:** Facilitate opportunities for neurodiverse individuals to connect with peers who share similar experiences. Peer support and advocacy groups can provide a sense of belonging, understanding, and empowerment.

6. **Celebrate neurodiverse achievements:** Recognize and celebrate the achievements and contributions of neurodiverse individuals in various domains, such as academics, arts, sciences, or sports. This helps shift the focus from deficits to abilities.

Creating Supportive Environments at Home, School, and Work

Creating supportive environments is essential for the well-being and success of neurodiverse individuals. Whether it's at home, school, or work, providing a nurturing and accommodating environment can help individuals thrive. Here are strategies for creating supportive environments:

1. **Clear communication:** Use clear and concise communication strategies that are tailored to the individual's needs and preferences. Provide instructions, expectations, and feedback in a way that is easily understood.

2. **Establish routines and structure:** Create predictable routines and structures to provide a sense of stability and reduce anxiety. Visual supports, such as schedules or checklists, can

help individuals navigate daily activities and transitions.

3. **Individualized accommodations:** Identify and implement individualized accommodations that support the specific needs of neurodiverse individuals. These accommodations may include preferential seating, extra time for tasks, access to assistive technologies, or modified assignments.

4. **Positive behavior support:** Implement positive behavior support strategies to encourage desired behaviors and address challenging behaviors. This may involve using visual cues, rewards systems, or teaching alternative coping strategies.

5. **Collaboration and teamwork:** Foster collaboration and teamwork among family members, educators, and colleagues. Encourage open communication, sharing of ideas, and collective problem-solving to create a supportive network.

6. **Sensory considerations:** Take into account sensory sensitivities and provide an environment that minimizes sensory overload. This can involve creating quiet spaces, offering noise-canceling headphones, or allowing sensory breaks.

7. **Professional development:** Provide ongoing professional development and training to educators, employers, and support staff. This ensures they have the knowledge and skills to effectively support neurodiverse individuals.

Advocacy and Raising Awareness

Advocacy plays a vital role in ensuring that the rights and needs of neurodiverse individuals are recognized and met. By advocating for inclusive policies and raising awareness, we can drive positive change and create a more inclusive society. Here are strategies for advocacy and raising awareness:

1. **Promote self-advocacy:** Encourage neurodiverse individuals to develop self-advocacy skills and empower them to voice their needs and preferences. Provide support and resources to enhance their ability to advocate for themselves.

2. **Engage in community outreach:** Reach out to community organizations, schools, workplaces, and government agencies to raise awareness about neurodiversity. Organize workshops, seminars, or awareness campaigns to share information and promote understanding.

3. **Collaborate with advocacy groups:** Collaborate with local and national advocacy groups that focus on neurodiversity. Join forces to advocate for policy changes, improved support services, and increased inclusivity in various domains.

4. **Support legislation and policies:** Stay informed about legislative initiatives related to neurodiversity and advocate for policies that promote inclusivity, accessibility, and equal rights. Write letters to policymakers or participate in advocacy campaigns to support these initiatives.

5. **Share personal stories:** Encourage individuals and families affected by neurodiversity to share their personal stories. Personal narratives can be powerful tools for raising awareness, challenging misconceptions, and fostering empathy.

6. **Engage in social media activism:** Utilize social media platforms to raise awareness about neurodiversity, share educational resources, and challenge stigma and misconceptions. Use hashtags and participate in online discussions to amplify voices and advocate for change.

Addressing Stigma and Misconceptions

Addressing stigma and misconceptions associated with neurodiversity is crucial for creating a more inclusive and accepting society. Stigma can lead to discrimination, social exclusion, and hinder access to necessary support and resources. Here are strategies for addressing stigma and misconceptions:

1. **Education and dispelling myths:** Provide accurate information about neurodiversity through educational initiatives, workshops, and community discussions. Challenge common myths and misconceptions by presenting scientific evidence and personal experiences.

2. **Promote positive language:** Encourage the use of person-first language that emphasizes the individual rather than their diagnosis. Language choices can have a significant impact on

how neurodiverse individuals are perceived and treated.

3. **Media representation:** Advocate for accurate and positive representation of neurodiverse individuals in the media. Encourage media outlets to portray diverse characters and storylines that challenge stereotypes and promote understanding.

4. **Promote empathy and understanding:** Foster empathy and understanding by encouraging open dialogue and promoting personal connections. Encourage individuals to listen to the experiences and perspectives of neurodiverse individuals and challenge their preconceived notions.

5. **Create safe spaces:** Establish safe spaces where neurodiverse individuals can feel accepted, supported, and free from judgment. This can include support groups, community centers, or online platforms that provide a sense of belonging.

6. **Lead by example:** Model inclusive and accepting behavior in personal interactions and advocate for inclusive practices within organizations and institutions. By demonstrating acceptance and respect, we can inspire others to do the same.

Addressing stigma and misconceptions requires a collective effort from individuals, communities, and institutions. By challenging stereotypes, promoting understanding, and fostering inclusivity, we can create a society that embraces and celebrates neurodiversity.

FUTURE

DIRECTIONS

AND EMERGING

RESEARCH

Latest Advancements in ADHD
and Autism Research

Research in the field of ADHD and Autism has been rapidly advancing, contributing to a deeper understanding of these conditions and leading to the development of new interventions and strategies. Here are some recent advancements in research:

1. **Genetic and molecular studies:** Advances in genetic and molecular research have identified specific genes and genetic variations associated with ADHD and Autism. This knowledge helps in understanding the underlying biological mechanisms and can potentially lead to targeted

treatments and interventions.

2. **Brain imaging and neurobiology:** Neuroimaging techniques, such as functional magnetic resonance imaging (fMRI) and electroencephalography (EEG), have provided insights into the structural and functional differences in the brains of individuals with ADHD and Autism. These findings contribute to understanding the neural basis of these conditions and inform the development of interventions.

3. **Early detection and intervention:** Research has emphasized the importance of early detection and intervention for better outcomes in ADHD and Autism. Studies have focused on identifying early markers and developing screening tools to enable early identification and intervention, promoting improved developmental trajectories.

4. **Environmental risk factors:** Research has explored various environmental factors that may contribute to the development of ADHD and Autism. These include prenatal and perinatal factors, exposure to certain toxins, and socio-environmental influences. Understanding these risk factors helps in implementing preventive measures and interventions.

5. **Co-occurring conditions:** Studies have shed light on the high rates of co-occurring conditions in individuals with ADHD and Autism. Research has explored the connections between these conditions and their impact on diagnosis, treatment, and outcomes. This knowledge

aids in developing comprehensive and tailored interventions.

6. **Personalized medicine approaches:** Research is focusing on the development of personalized medicine approaches for ADHD and Autism. By considering an individual's unique genetic and neurobiological profile, treatment strategies can be tailored to their specific needs, maximizing effectiveness and minimizing side effects.

Promising Treatment Approaches and Therapies

Advancements in research have led to the emergence of promising treatment approaches and therapies for individuals with ADHD and Autism. Here are some notable interventions:

1. **Behavioral interventions:** Behavioral interventions, such as Applied Behavior Analysis (ABA), have shown efficacy in addressing challenging behaviors and promoting skill development in individuals with ADHD and Autism. These interventions focus on reinforcing positive behaviors and providing structured supports.

2. **Social skills training:** Social skills training programs aim to enhance social interaction and communication skills in individuals with ADHD and Autism. These programs provide explicit instruction, role-playing, and practice

opportunities to improve social understanding and interaction.

3. **Cognitive-behavioral therapy (CBT):** CBT is a therapeutic approach that targets cognitive processes and behavioral patterns. It has been adapted for individuals with ADHD and Autism to address challenges such as impulsivity, emotional regulation, and executive functioning difficulties.

4. **Medication:** Medication continues to play a significant role in the treatment of ADHD, with stimulant and non-stimulant medications being commonly prescribed. For Autism, medication may be used to manage specific symptoms or co-occurring conditions, such as attention difficulties or anxiety.

5. **Parent training programs:** Parent training programs provide parents with strategies and skills to effectively manage their child's behaviors and support their development. These programs empower parents and caregivers to create structured and supportive home environments.

6. **Multimodal interventions:** Multimodal interventions combine different approaches, such as behavioral interventions, social skills training, and medication, to address the diverse needs of individuals with ADHD and Autism. These comprehensive approaches recognize the multifaceted nature of these conditions and aim for holistic support.

It's important to note that treatment approaches

should be individualized, considering the unique strengths, challenges, and preferences of each individual. Collaborative decision-making involving healthcare professionals, individuals, and families is essential in determining the most suitable interventions.

Technological Innovations and Assistive Devices

Technological advancements have brought about innovative tools and assistive devices that can significantly benefit individuals with ADHD and Autism. These technologies aim to enhance communication, learning, organization, and overall well-being. Here are some examples:

1. **Augmentative and alternative communication (AAC) devices:** AAC devices enable individuals with communication difficulties to express themselves effectively. These devices range from picture-based communication systems to speech-generating devices that convert symbols or text into speech.

2. **Wearable technology:** Wearable devices, such as smartwatches and activity trackers, can assist individuals with ADHD and Autism in various ways. They can provide reminders, timers, and visual schedules, promoting organization and

time management skills.

3. **Virtual reality (VR) therapy:** VR therapy is being explored as a therapeutic tool for individuals with ADHD and Autism. It provides immersive and controlled environments for practicing social skills, managing sensory sensitivities, and addressing anxiety in a safe and controlled manner.

4. **Mobile applications (apps):** There is a wide range of apps available for smartphones and tablets that cater to the needs of individuals with ADHD and Autism. These apps can assist with organization, task management, self-regulation, and social skill development.

5. **Sensory aids:** Sensory aids, such as noise-canceling headphones or weighted blankets, can help individuals with sensory sensitivities to manage their environments and reduce sensory overload. These aids promote comfort, focus, and self-regulation.

6. **Assistive technology for learning:** Assistive technology tools, such as text-to-speech software, word prediction programs, or graphic organizers, support individuals with ADHD and Autism in their academic pursuits. These tools facilitate information processing, reading comprehension, and written expression.

Technological innovations continue to advance rapidly, offering new possibilities for supporting individuals with ADHD and Autism. It's important to consider individual needs and preferences when selecting and implementing assistive devices and technologies.

The Role of Neurodivergent Individuals in Shaping the Future

Neurodivergent individuals have a significant role to play in shaping a more inclusive and accommodating future. Their unique perspectives, strengths, and talents bring valuable contributions to various domains, including education, employment, technology, and the arts. Here are some aspects highlighting their role:

1. **Advocacy and self-advocacy:** Neurodivergent individuals are at the forefront of advocacy efforts, promoting awareness, acceptance, and equal rights. Their voices and personal experiences are instrumental in challenging stereotypes, addressing stigma, and driving positive change.

2. **Innovation and creativity:** Many neurodivergent individuals possess exceptional creativity, innovative thinking, and problem-solving skills. Their unique perspectives can lead to breakthroughs in various fields, contributing to scientific advancements, technological innovations, and artistic expression.

3. **Diverse talents and strengths:** Neurodivergent individuals often exhibit a wide range of talents

and strengths, such as attention to detail, pattern recognition, exceptional memory, or intense focus. These abilities can be harnessed and valued in workplaces, educational settings, and creative endeavors.

4. **Inclusive design and accessibility:** Neurodivergent individuals bring firsthand knowledge and insights into the design of inclusive environments, products, and services. Their input is invaluable in creating spaces and technologies that accommodate diverse sensory, cognitive, and social needs.

5. **Empathy and understanding:** Neurodivergent individuals often have a deep empathy and understanding of the challenges faced by others. Their lived experiences can foster empathy, compassion, and a sense of social responsibility, promoting a more caring and inclusive society.

6. **Peer support and mentoring:** Neurodivergent individuals can provide peer support and mentoring to others facing similar challenges. Their experiences, strategies, and successes can inspire and guide others in their journey towards self-acceptance, personal growth, and achievement.

It is essential to involve neurodivergent individuals in decision-making processes and provide opportunities for their meaningful participation. By embracing their unique perspectives and strengths, we can create a future that celebrates diversity, inclusivity, and equal opportunities for all.

CONCLUSION

Recap of Key Points Covered in the Guide

Throughout this guide, we have explored various aspects of ADHD and Autism, aiming to provide a comprehensive understanding and practical strategies for managing these conditions. Let's recap some of the key points covered:

1. ADHD and Autism are neurodevelopmental conditions that affect individuals in different ways, impacting their attention, social interaction, communication, and behavior.

2. Understanding and managing these conditions is crucial for individuals, families, educators, and communities to provide appropriate support and promote positive outcomes.

3. There are similarities and differences between ADHD and Autism, and it is not uncommon for individuals to have both conditions simultaneously. Accurate diagnosis and differentiation can be challenging but are essential for effective intervention.

4. Early intervention and support play a significant role in improving outcomes for individuals with ADHD and Autism. Identifying and addressing their specific needs early on can lead to better development and adaptation.

5. Various interventions and therapies are available to support individuals with ADHD and Autism. These include behavioral and educational interventions, medication options, supportive therapies, and individualized accommodations.

6. Creating supportive environments at home, school, and work is essential for individuals with ADHD and Autism. Understanding their unique challenges, providing accommodations, and fostering inclusivity can help them thrive.

7. Advocacy, raising awareness, and addressing stigma are crucial for creating an inclusive society that embraces neurodiversity. Promoting acceptance, understanding, and access to support and resources is vital for the well-being of individuals with ADHD and Autism.

8. Research and advancements in the field are continually expanding our knowledge and leading to promising treatment approaches, technological innovations, and assistive devices.

Encouragement and Hope for Individuals with ADHD and Autism

To individuals with ADHD and Autism, it is essential to remember that you are not defined by your diagnosis. You have unique strengths, talents, and perspectives that contribute to the world in meaningful ways. While you may face challenges, know that you are not alone, and there is support available to help you navigate your journey. Embrace your strengths, celebrate your successes, and remember that growth and progress are possible.

Seek out a network of support, including family, friends, healthcare professionals, and support groups. Surround yourself with people who understand and accept you for who you are. Remember to take care of yourself, prioritize your well-being, and practice self-compassion. You are deserving of love, understanding, and support.

It's important to set realistic goals, break tasks into manageable steps, and celebrate your achievements along the way. Remember that progress may be non-linear, and setbacks are a natural part of the journey. Be patient with yourself and keep moving forward. You have the resilience and strength to overcome challenges and reach your full potential.

Final Words of Support and Encouragement

In closing, we want to express our support and encouragement to all individuals with ADHD and Autism, their families, and their support networks. Remember that understanding, acceptance, and appropriate support are key ingredients in promoting well-being and success.

Each person's journey is unique, and there is no one-size-fits-all approach. Embrace your individuality, advocate for your needs, and surround yourself with a community that uplifts and empowers you. You have the ability to create positive change, not only in your own life but also in the lives of others.

Never forget that you are capable, resilient, and deserving of happiness and fulfillment. Your unique perspectives, talents, and strengths can contribute to a world that values diversity and inclusivity. Keep pushing forward, and believe in your potential. You are not alone on this journey, and together, we can create a more inclusive and understanding society.

Wishing you all the best in your endeavors and a future filled with growth, support, and meaningful connections.